PRAYER &

THE MASTER KEY
to the
IMPOSSIBLE

by Gordon Lindsay

Published By
CHRIST FOR THE NATIONS INC.
P.O. Box 769000
Dallas, TX 75376-9000

First Printing – 1974
Reprints – 1974, 1975, 1976, 1977, 1979, 1981,
1983, 1986, 1989, 1991, 1994, 1996, 1998
Fourteenth Reprint – 2000

TABLE OF CONTENTS

All Scripture NKJV unless otherwise noted.

Chapter 1

Prayer & Fasting — Master Key To The Impossible

Adam and Eve's disobedience by eating the forbidden fruit was the original cause of man's losing his God-given dominion in the Garden of Eden. Christ made possible the restoration of man's dominion by fasting forty days and nights in the wilderness, overcoming the fiercest attacks of the enemy (Lk. 4:1-13).

Adam and Eve were given the Garden of Eden as their home, with instructions that they might partake freely of the fruit in the Garden — except the tree of knowledge of good and evil. But Eve saw that "the tree was good for food, that it was pleasant to the eyes" (Gen. 3:6). She took some and ate, along with her husband, Adam. Thereby Adam and Eve ushered sin and sorrow into the world for themselves and their descendants.

Christ, the Second Adam, refused to give in to temptation. Rather than create and eat bread at the devil's suggestion, He completed His fast, winning back that which was lost by Adam and Eve. As we will see, prayer and fasting was the master key that Christ used to make the impossible possible. This master key can be used by you and me to meet the desperate needs of humanity and make the impossible become possible.

ESAU SOLD HIS BIRTHRIGHT
FOR A POT OF STEW

It is true that a lack of discipline over the appetites of the flesh leads to spiritual barrenness and even disaster. Fasting, denying oneself food, has the opposite effect: It gives men a new grip on God. Esau's downfall was similar to Adam and Eve's: He sold his birthright for a bite of food.

Esau was the elder of twins; rightfully, the inheritance belonged to him. He could have been the father of the chosen race instead of Jacob. But there was one fundamental difference between the brothers. Jacob had faith and prized the birthright. Esau thought only in earthly terms. In a moment of temptation, he gave up his birthright for a mere pot of stew.

> And Jacob said, "Sell me this day thy birthright." And Esau said, "Behold I am at the point to die: and what profit shall this birthright do to me?" And Jacob said, "Swear to me this day"; and he sware unto him: and he sold his birthright unto Jacob (Gen. 25:31-33).

By gratifying his appetite that day, Esau forfeited the glory that could have been his. And when he later became remorseful for his act, he was not repentant.

Fasting reverses the order. The discipline of the soul that comes from abstaining from the earthly opens the door to the heavenly. Again and again in Scripture, we find people losing their place with God through failure to control the appetites of the flesh. At the same time, we find examples of others who, through the discipline of fasting, overcame all obstacles and obtained answers from God that changed the destiny of kingdoms.

By lusting for the delicacies of Egypt, the Israelites lost the blessing of God. They "lusted exceedingly in the wilderness, and tested God in the desert. And he gave them their request, but sent leanness into their soul" (Psa. 106:14,15). But their leader, Moses, by his intercession and his fast of forty days, saved them from destruction as a nation.

Those living in Noah's day were so given over to satisfying their physical appetites, they were unaware of the gathering clouds of judgment until suddenly they found themselves being carried away in the Flood.

> But as the days of Noah were, so also will the coming of the Son of Man be. For as in the days that were before the flood they were eating and drinking, marrying and giving in marriage, until the day that Noah entered into the ark (Matt. 24:37,38).

Christ warned His disciples not to be like those who lived in the days of Noah. He told them that through fasting and prayer they would be able to overcome the powers of evil, cast out demons and move mountains.

> Assuredly, I say to you, if you have faith as a mustard seed, you will say to this mountain, "Move from here to there," and it will move; and nothing will be impossible for you. However, this kind does not go out except by prayer and fasting (Matt. 17:20,21).

In this way Christ showed that prayer and fasting was the master key to change the impossible to the possible.

Daniel 5 tells us that one night King Belshazzar of Babylon indulged in a great banquet, in which he and a thousand noblemen feasted and drank wine together. In their drunken revelry, they profaned the gold and silver cups that Belshazzar's father, Nebuchadnezzar, had stolen from the Temple in Jerusalem. But even as they did, a human hand appeared and began writing on the wall. That same night Belshazzar was slain. Daniel, the man of God who interpreted the handwriting, was the one who had fasted twenty-one days until the power of the prince of the kingdom of darkness was broken and deliverance came to his nation. This prophet knew the key to victory was fasting prayer.

Of John the Baptist, Jesus said there was none greater born of woman. By his life of self-denial, he prepared for the coming of the Messiah.

Fasting will win the battle and put the enemy to flight, even though failures in the past have been many. When Israel lost two great battles and was humbled to the dust by the tragic loss of thousands of lives, her people fasted and wept before the Lord. The next day defeat was turned into victory (Judg. 20).

Jezebel fed the prophets of Baal from her sumptuous table. But through Elijah, the prophet of God, they came under the judgment of God. Elijah then had to flee from the wrath of Jezebel. He fasted forty days as he walked to Mt. Horeb where he heard "a still small voice" (I Ki. 19:12). He left there under a mighty anointing of God and returned to Israel to execute the judgments of the Lord. Never again did he flee from man or woman. Faith so dominated his being that even death could not master him, and he was taken up by a chariot of fire into heaven.

The prophet Jonah warned the residents of Nineveh that in 40 days their city was to be destroyed. The king and the people heeded the warning. They put on sackcloth and fell on their faces in fasting and repentance. The city, with a population of 160,000, was saved.

In the days of Esther, all hope seemed gone for the Jews. The king had signed a document giving the evil prime minister, Haman, and his men the authority to destroy all of that race. But Queen Esther, her maidens and Mordecai fasted three days and three nights. Then, risking her own life, Esther made a petition before the king. Not only were her people saved, but Haman was hanged on the same gallows he had made for Mordecai.

Ezra had a commission from the king to carry the gold and silver of the temple back to Jerusalem. He knew he must travel through country infested with thieves and robbers to whom the gold would be a rich prize. Ezra and his companions fasted and prayed, and God took them safely to their destination.

At one point in history, the Philistines humbled the Israelites by a great defeat. They had even taken the Ark of God. It seemed that Israel no longer had the power to stand against this fierce enemy. Then Samuel and the people cried to God and fasted. The Lord came on the scene with a great thunder, scattering the enemy. The Philistines' defeat was so overwhelming that they did not come against Israel again during the days of Samuel's leadership.

Paul, a persecutor of Christians, met the Lord on the Damascus road. Blinded by the vision, he was led into the city where for three days he prayed and fasted. Then God told Ananias to go to Paul and to lay hands on him so that he could receive his sight and be filled with the Holy Spirit. From that experience, Paul went forward to become the greatest apostle of all.

For long centuries the gentiles had been excluded from the commonwealth of Israel and all its blessings. But a man by the name of Cornelius fasted, prayed and gave alms to the poor. As a result, an angel came to him and told him to send for Peter. At the same time the Lord gave a vision to Peter and showed him that the gentiles were no more unclean, but were to receive the Gospel the same as Israel.

As a prisoner, Paul was taken on board ship. The captain, disregarding the divine warning given by the apostle, put out to sea. As Paul had forewarned, they ran into a storm. It continued for fourteen days and nights. It would have no doubt taken the lives of all on board except that during that time, Paul and the crew fasted. On the fourteenth day the answer came. All 276 people on board were saved. Fasting and prayer triumphed over the destructive forces of the elements!

The biblical examples are many. When all else failed, fasting and prayer turned the tide. It is true that prayer changes things. But of all prayers, the fasting prayer has the greatest effect of all. Yes, it is the master key to making the impossible possible.

Chapter 2

Important Facts About Fasting

There are a number of important facts that everyone should know about fasting. For one thing, the Bible speaks of three kinds of fasts. The first is supernatural fasting — without either food or water. The second is ordinary fasting — no food is eaten, but water is taken to replenish what is lost. The third kind of fasting is mentioned by Daniel; he ate "no pleaseant food."

THE SUPERNATURAL FAST

This supernatural fast occurred in the ministry of Moses on Mount Sinai when he went the second time to receive the Ten Commandments, after he had interceded for his nation. This fasting of Moses resulted in the giving of the Mosaic covenant to Israel.

> Then the LORD said to Moses, "Write these words, for according to the tenor of these words I have made a covenant with you and with Israel." So he was there with the LORD forty days and forty nights; he neither ate bread nor drank water. And He wrote on the tablets the words of the covenant, the Ten Commandments (Ex.34:27,28).

In the natural, man can fast only a very few days without food or water, and this certainly should never be attempted for any length of time unless divinely directed. Moses' case was a special one of supernatural character and was associated with a biblical event of dispensational importance. During those days, God's power came upon Moses so that even his face shown with the transfiguring glory of God (Ex. 34:35). The Lord had placed Moses in a cleft of a rock as He passed by. The glory of God's presence was so intense that Moses would have perished had not God supernaturally protected him (Ex. 33:20-23).

While it is possible that Christ fasted without water during His forty days in the wilderness, there is no Scriptural record to that effect. Fasting without water, except for very short periods (such as Esther's fast), is not the kind of fasting generally taught in Scripture.

FASTING WITHOUT FOOD BUT DRINKING WATER — THE TOTAL FAST

Ordinary fasting includes drinking of water, for water is not a food. Water is an important element in the body, but it contains no calories or nutrition of any kind. Since the body is 80% water and may lose several quarts daily, to maintain a temperature equilibrium in the body, water is very essential to life. It must be constantly replenished in the human system. The total fast excludes the eating of food, but does include the drinking of water.

For those who enter the total fast, remember this: Such a fast must be broken slowly. The first day or two, only diluted juices should be taken. Then add light fruit for a few days. After that, the diet may gradually include heavier foods. To eat a heavy meal after a long fast is to invite serious trouble.

If at the end of the first day of a fast, one feels enervating weakness and/or a strong hunger, it may be advisable for him to take a small amount of nourishment. By the second or third day, the feeling of hunger will have gradually diminished and the weakness will not be so pronounced. Just as the body needs to adjust gradually when a fast is over, so there is the need of adjustment while entering into a fast. The requirements of individuals vary. Each one should learn how he can most easily enter into a fast with a minimum of physical and mental weakness.

THIRD KIND OF FAST — "NO PLEASANT FOOD"

About a certain fast, Daniel the prophet says: "I ate no pleasant food, no meat or wine came into my mouth" (Dan. 10:3). He did not refrain from eating altogether, but ate "no pleasant food." The word *pleasant* in the Hebrew is "chamadoth." Moffat's translation says, "I ate not delicacies." Exactly what he may have eaten, we do not know. It probably was very little, although this was not a total fast.

Some who teach on fasting consider only the total fast, which many Christians have neither the faith nor physical fortitude to undergo. They attempt fasting, but become so weak that they are unable to continue. Or if they do continue, they are unable to pray effectively with the result that they experience defeat instead of victory.

THE NON-TOTAL FAST

What we have to say at this point does not apply to those who are able to fast totally. God bless them, and may the Lord lead them in more such fasts. But what we are interested in is helping the thousands of people who so far have found it impossible to fast, or who at least do not fast, yet face battles which can only be won by prayer and fasting.

One problem for many is that they must continue their daily work while fasting. They realize it would be best to suspend their regular duties until after the fast, but it is impossible for them to do so.

What is a non-total fast? Simply this: Drinking juices — orange, tomato, pineapple, etc. Since juices have very few calories, drinking only juices permits the system to get into the true state of a fast — an absence of hunger. But at the same time, minerals and vitamins continue to be supplied to the body. The stomach is quiet and there is little of the nausea and weakness many experience in a total fast. The juices supply sufficient strength to pray and seek God, which is crucial. It is better to drink juices while fasting and have the strength to pray and battle the enemy than to try a total fast and be nauseous much of the time and have no strength to pray. Also, a fruit juice fast can be broken in a short time, whereas the total fast requires days.

We recommend that one drink only a small amount of juice at a time. Whenever there is weakness or nausea, he should take a little juice, preferably by sipping. A hot drink not prepared with milk may be drunk occasionally.

It is important for the person who is fasting to give much time to prayer. This is the time to literally "pray without ceasing," though not necessarily in audible prayer all the time. But gradually the spirit of intercession should become as natural as breathing.

Chapter 3

Right & Wrong Ways to Fast

Just as there is a right way to pray, a right way to worship God and a right way to exercise the gifts of the Spirit, so there is a right way to fast. Great results may be obtained through fasting and prayer, but it is possible to fast in a way that will do more harm than good. It is important that we avoid those things that might lead to such consequences.

FASTING TO BE DONE IN SECRET AS MUCH AS POSSIBLE

The right method of fasting is so important that Christ called attention to it at the beginning of His ministry. Later, He showed His disciples the power in fasting — that it could result in faith that would move mountains and cast out the most powerful demons (Matt. 17:20,21). But in His first lesson on fasting, He showed how fasting could be used to exalt oneself. He called attention to the Pharisees, who let everyone know they were fasting so they would be honored. Jesus warned against this:

> Moreover, when you fast, do not be like the hypocrites, with a sad countenance. For they disfigure their faces that they may appear to men to be fasting. Assuredly, I say to you, they have their reward. But you, when you

fast, anoint your head and wash your face, so that you do not appear to men to be fasting, but to your Father who is in the secret place; and your Father who sees in secret will reward you openly (Matt. 6:16-18).

It is vain to fast to receive the honor of men. God has a place for each member of His body. One must seek to fulfill the purpose that God intended for him. Only then will he find permanent peace of mind and soul. It is wrong to fast to seek power merely to gratify human ambition. "For exaltation comes neither from the east nor from the west nor from the south" (Psa. 75:6). It comes from the Lord. To gain power with God, his motive must be pure. His desire must spring from compassion for suffering humanity who need deliverance from sin, sickness, evil habits and the oppression of Satan.

It is best to keep the fact that one is on a fast as quiet as possible. But there is no need to be under bondage about it. The proper attitude is to be indifferent as to whether others know you are fasting or not. Your own family, of course, will be sure to know if you are fasting. Then there are times when many fast together.

There was a Pharisee who boasted of his fasting. This proud ritualist looked with scorn on the penitent tax collector who was confessing his sins, while to himself he boasted of his own deeds, which included fasting twice a week.

The Pharisee stood and prayed thus with himself, "God, I thank You that I am not like this ... tax collector. I fast twice a week; I give tithes of all that I possess." And the tax collector, standing afar off, would not so much as raise his eyes to heaven, but beat his breast, saying, "God be merciful to me a sinner!" I tell you, this man went down to his house justified rather than the other; for everyone who exalts himself will be abased, and he who humbles himself will be exalted (Lk. 18:11-14).

FASTING AND SELFISHNESS DON'T MIX

In Isaiah 58 we read how the fasting by religious people of Isaiah's day originated in selfishness. They had no thought of humbling themselves before God. They just wanted secure benefits which would give them a competitive advantage over others. There are always those who fast in order to secure personal power. Others fast for aesthetic reasons. Still others may fast for health purposes. Moslems fast for religious reasons, even though they do not believe in the divinity of Christ. Hindus fast in the practice of their mystical arts. None of these cases can be considered biblical fasting, nor can divine blessing be poured out on the devotees of false religions.

Fasting is absolutely of no benefit to those who are not walking in obedience to God.

> Thus says the LORD to this people: "Thus they have loved to wander; they have not restrained their feet. Therefore the LORD does not accept them; He will remember their iniquity now, and punish their sins." Then the LORD said to me, "Do not pray for this people, for their good. When they fast, I will not hear their cry; and when they offer burnt offering and grain offering, I will not accept them. But I will consume them by the sword, by the famine, and by the pestilence" (Jer. 14:10-12).

As great a man as David was, he committed an evil that even fasting and prayer could not fully repair. He deliberately committed adultery with Bathsheba, and then arranged for the death of her husband, Uriah. The child born of this union became deathly sick. David, overcome with remorse, fasted and prayed for seven days, but the child died.

GOD RECOGNIZES HUMILITY, REPENTANCE AND SINCERITY OF HEART

Fasting is the master key by which the impossible becomes

possible. But humility, repentance and sincerity of heart are the keys to the type of fasting recognized by God.

Chapter 4

Prayer & Fasting That Saved Over Two Million Lives

"So he was there with the Lord forty days and forty nights; he neither ate bread nor drank water. And He wrote upon the tablets the words of the covenant, the Ten Commandments" (Ex. 34:28).

When Moses came down from Mount Sinai, he was met with the greatest crisis of his life. During his absence, catastrophic events had developed in the camp of Israel. In order to understand the magnitude of the crisis that confronted Moses, let us rehearse briefly the events prior to this crisis.

Forty years before, Moses had felt God's call to deliver his brethren. In those days, human ambition burned within him and he attempted to accomplish God's work in his own power. He failed miserably and was forced to flee to the desert. For forty years he tended sheep for his father-in-law while his ambitions faded and were almost forgotten. He desired only to live out the balance of his days in peace.

But God would not have it so. Though Moses did not realize it, he was at last ready to fulfill the calling of God and enter into the ministry the Lord had ordained for him.

Now the man Moses was very humble, more than all
men who were on the face of the earth (Num. 12:3).
It is only when we have reached a place of deep humility that we
are in a position to accomplish a great work for God. At the burning
bush, God commissioned Moses to lead the children of Israel out of
Egyptian bondage and into the Promised Land. This commission
was accompanied by an awesome series of signs, wonders and
judgments. Afterward, Moses obtained a release from Pharaoh to
take his people out of Egypt. The Israelites crossed the Red Sea
through supernatural intervention. Then Moses held out his rod and
the sea returned to its place, swallowing up Pharaoh and his chariots.

On the other side of the sea, the Lord began to deal with Israel
as His redeemed people, making a special covenant with them and
promising that if they kept it, they would become His "peculiar
treasure," a kingdom of priests:

Now therefore, if you will indeed obey My voice and
keep My covenant, then you shall be a special treasure
to Me above all people; for all the earth is Mine. And
you shall be to Me a kingdom of priests and a holy nation
(Ex. 19:5,6).

Moses presented this covenant to Israel and the people agreed to
its terms:

Then all the people answered together and said, "All that
the LORD has spoken we will do" (Ex. 19:8).

Then Moses returned to the mountain to receive the provisions
of the covenant in detail. This required several weeks of time.
Unfortunately, as Moses' time with God was coming to an end,
something terrible was happening among the people of Israel. Some
of the more impetuous ones, seeing that Moses had been delayed in
coming down the mountain, considered it an opportunity to subvert
Israel to their own evil designs. They persuaded Aaron to consent
to make a golden calf, and then said to the people, "This is your god,
O Israel, that brought you out of the land of Egypt" (Ex. 32:4).

Up on the mountain, God revealed to Moses what had taken place in the camp. After all the signs and miracles He had performed before their very eyes, they had taken part in this act of inexcusable rebellion — an effrontery to God. The people had rejected Jehovah and turned to gods made by their own hands.

> And the LORD said to Moses, "I have seen this people, and indeed it is a stiff-necked people! Now therefore, let Me alone, that My wrath may burn hot against them and I may consume them. And I will make of you a great nation" (Ex. 32:9,10).

When Moses came down from the mountain, he soon learned the horrible details. Not only had the golden calf been made, but the people had been drawn into an orgy of licentious worship of it, even to dancing in the nude. In his anger, Moses broke the tablets of the commandments and sent orders for the execution of the leaders of the rebellion.

THE PRAYER AND FASTING OF MOSES

Moses was face to face with the greatest crisis of his life. He returned to the mountain, resolved that he would neither eat nor drink until God brought a solution. He knew that he must prevail with God. For nearly six weeks Moses fasted on the Mount of God:

> So he was there with the LORD forty days and forty nights; he neither ate bread nor drank water. And He wrote on the tablets the words of the covenant, the Ten Commandments (Ex. 34:28).

There on the mountain, God gave Moses the opportunity to become the progenitor of a great nation. He said, "Let me alone, that ... I may consume them. And I will make of you a great nation" (Ex. 32:10). To someone else, this would have been a great temptation. It was an offer which no doubt would have been accepted by a person of lesser stature. But not Moses. He was not thinking of personal ambitions, but of the millions of people about to die under the judgment of God. He interceded before God in agony of soul. He called the Lord's attention to the fact that if Israel perished in the wilderness, the heathen would say that God brought them out into the wilderness to destroy them. "Turn from Your fierce wrath, and relent from this harm to Your people" (Ex. 32:12), interceded the prophet. He mentioned God's promises — His covenant with Abraham (vs. 13). In this way, Moses prevailed! For "the LORD relented from the harm which He said He would do to His people" (vs. 14). Moses put the master key to work, and he obtained results.

DIVINE FORGIVENESS FOR ISRAEL

Moses' intercession spared the people of Israel extinction as a nation. But the prophet was not satisfied. He wanted forgiveness for the people. The next day, after conferring with the children of Israel and calling them to repent of their sin, he again fell on his face before God. He asked God not only to spare the Israelites, but to forgive them. If God would not forgive Israel, Moses asked that he too be blotted out of God's book. Moved by such selflessness, God reassured him: He would never blot out the name of His faithful ones, but only those who sinned against Him.

Yet now, if You will forgive their sin — but if not, I pray, blot me out of Your book which You have written. And the LORD said to Moses, "Whoever has sinned against Me, I will blot him out of My book" (Ex. 32:32,33).

Now Moses entered into his third intercession. It was not enough that God send an angel before him into the Promised Land. Moses would not go with this people unless the very presence of God went also.

And He said, "My Presence will go with you, and I will give you rest." Then he said to Him, "If Your Presence does not go with us, do not bring us up from here" (Ex. 33:14,15).

Again Moses prevailed with God! The Lord agreed to go with Moses and the people on their journey to the Promised Land.

MOSES ASKS GOD TO SHOW HIM HIS GLORY

In the course of the intercession, Moses had drawn very near to God. While he was experiencing this wonderful visitation of divine presence, Moses asked God for the privilege of witnessing His glory. And again his prayer was answered! God hid him in a cleft of a rock, and let him behold a vision of His glory!

> And the LORD said, "Here is a place by Me, and you shall stand on the rock. So it shall be, while My glory passes by, that I will put you in the cleft of the rock, and will cover you with My hand while I pass by" (Ex. 33:21,22).

The bridge that had broken down had been rebuilt. The breach that could have spelled eternal doom for millions had been restored. Broken communion had been renewed. For forty days and nights Moses was on his face before God. There God gave him new tablets of stone. And there He renewed His promise to drive out the Canaanites and give Israel the land flowing with milk and honey.

> And He said: "Behold, I make a covenant. Before all your people I will do marvels such as have not been done in all the earth, nor in any nation; and all the people among whom you are shall see the work of the LORD. For it is an awesome thing that I will do with you" (Ex. 34:10).

AFTERMATH OF THE FORTY DAYS OF FASTING

At the end of forty days, Moses came down from the mountain. The glory of God was upon him. His face glowed so that the Children of Israel could not look at him. In fact, he was compelled to wear a veil over his face.

> And whenever the children of Israel saw the face of Moses, that the skin of Moses' face shone, then Moses would put the veil on his face again, until he went in to speak with Him (Ex. 34:35).

MOSES' 40 DAYS WITH GOD MADE THE IMPOSSIBLE POSSIBLE

And so the restoration of Israel was completed. National redemption was ushered in because God had a man who was completely dedicated to Him. Those forty days and nights of prayer and fasting on Mount Horeb had broken off the powers of darkness and moved God's heart of compassion. Moses had received strength and vision for forty years in the wilderness that lay ahead. He had found the key that made the impossible possible, and he had not hesitated to use it.

Chapter 5

Fasting in the Old Testament

W e have seen the results of Moses' fasting on Mount Sinai. His intercessions and fasting for forty days saved the nation of Israel from perishing in the wilderness. We also saw that the ministry of intercession brought Moses into a high and honored position before the Lord. God unveiled His glory before him, a privilege never before accorded any mortal man.

But Moses was not the only one who achieved mighty results through fasting. Let us note some other great victories recorded in the Old Testament from fasting and prayer.

FASTING IN THE DAYS OF THE JUDGES

The days of the judges was a time of confusion in Israel, when "everyone did what was right in his own eyes" (Judg. 21:25). During this period, evil flourished. Finally, an act of such a revolting nature took place that even the dulled sensibilities of the nation were outraged. Action was taken to deal with the offenders. But the tribe of Benjamin took the side of those who committed the heinous crime, and prepared to defy Israel's demand. The Israelites sought the Lord in the matter, asking if they should use force to secure justice. God's answer was affirmative. However, though the Israelites were moving in the revealed will of God, the Benjamites succeeded in slaughtering some 40,000 people (Judg. 20:18-25) in two days of battle.

With this grave turn of events, the Israelites were really desperate. They sought God with prayer and fasting.

Then all the children of Israel, that is, all the people, went up and came to the house of God and wept. They sat there before the LORD and fasted that day until evening; and they offered burnt offerings and peace offerings before the LORD (Judg. 20:26).

Greatly humbled by these terrible reverses and by the number of lives that had been taken, they inquired of the Lord once more as to the proper course of action. This time the Lord not only gave them directions, but promised them victory which He had not done before. "And the Lord said, 'Go up, for tomorrow I will deliver them into your hand'" (Judg. 20:28).

The next day the Benjamites, cocksure because of their two previous victories, came against the children of Israel again. "But the Benjamites did not know that disaster was upon them. The LORD defeated Benjamin before Israel" (Judg. 20:34,35).

What are the lessons of this incident? The children of Israel had done right in seeking to avenge the awful deed of the men of Benjamin. They were obeying the Law of Moses, demanding that the offenders be punished. But they didn't take into account that lawlessness and evil had infiltrated Israel to the point that the powers of darkness had gained control. Their attempt to settle the matter purely through physical force resulted in failure and calamity to themselves. But when they sought the Lord in prayer and fasting, the powers of darkness were broken. God gave them victory, and the nation was purged of its awful sin. Fasting was the deciding factor in a grave situation. Israel had prayed twice, but only when they fasted along with their praying did deliverance come.

THE VICTORY OF JEHOSHAPHAT

Jehoshaphat was a godly king. He loved the Lord with all his heart. But he had one weakness: a tendency to make alliances with the ungodly, which got him into serious trouble more than once. But it was when a strong alliance of nations came against him that he met the greatest crisis of his life. Had divine intervention not come, his nation could have been destroyed.

Messengers came to King Jehoshaphat and told him that a powerful enemy was coming against him. It was no minor border skirmish, but a coalition of nations led by Israel's longtime enemies, Moab and Ammon, together with others from Syria. They were advancing rapidly toward Jerusalem with a large army. Jehoshaphat realized that the odds were stacked against him. In the natural, there was no way to avoid disaster. With the situation appearing hopeless, the king turned to God in prayer and fasting.

> And Jehoshaphat feared, and set himself to seek the LORD, and proclaimed a fast throughout all Judah. So Judah gathered together to ask help from the LORD; and from all the cities of Judah they came to seek the LORD (II Chr. 20:3,4).

Jehoshaphat not only fasted himself, but he gave orders for a fast to be observed throughout the land. People thronged into Jerusalem to join with the king in prayer and fasting. Their petition was led by the king (II Chr. 20:6-13). In this prayer, Jehoshaphat called God's attention to the covenants He had given to Abraham and Moses. He admitted his own powerlessness to stand before the enemy, and that his only hope was in God. Was this prayer that ascended to God from a fasting people answered? Yes indeed! A prophet, Jahaziel, was sent to them saying:

> Listen, all you of Judah and you inhabitants of Jerusalem, and you, King Jehoshaphat! Thus says the LORD to you: "Do not be afraid nor dismayed because of this great multitude, for the battle is not yours, but God's.

Tomorrow go down against them. ... You will not need to fight in this battle. Position yourselves, stand still and see the salvation of the LORD, who is with you, O Judah and Jerusalem!" Do not fear or be dismayed; tomorrow go out against them, for the LORD is with you (II Chr. 20:15-17).

Jahaziel gave certain instructions to the people. They were not to be discouraged or afraid to face this large army and the Lord would give them the victory — without any fighting! And so it was when they began to sing praises to the Lord, confusion came into the ranks of the enemy and they began to destroy one another until not one man was left. Judah returned to Jerusalem with joy, and the fear of God came on the nearby kingdoms (verses 27-29). Prayer and fasting saved the day.

ELIJAH AT HOREB

The prophet Elijah was one of the greatest Bible characters. The story of how he appeared before Ahab at the time of Israel's great apostasy is thrilling. His challenge of the Baal prophets and his calling down of fire from heaven turned the tide of apostasy. It brought the people to an open confession that the Lord was God. The subsequent prayer to break the drought and its remarkable answer is one of the most outstanding accounts in Scripture.

King Ahab told his wife Jezebel what Elijah had done and how he had put all the prophets of Baal to death. She sent a message to Elijah, threatening to take his life. Elijah's courage failed, and he fled for his life. Deep in the wilderness and far from his pursuers, he laid down under a juniper tree and asked the Lord to let him die. God did not answer this prayer, however, for He had other plans for the prophet. There under the tree, Elijah fell asleep. An angel woke him and told him to eat. He saw a loaf of bread and a jar of water. He ate and drank, then fell asleep. The angel woke him again and told him to get up and eat, or the trip would be too much for him.

A remarkable thing happened just before Elijah's protracted fast began. There is a preparation for a fast, even as there is a preparation of the heart for seeking God. Some rush into a fast on impulse rather than because of the moving of the Spirit. When Jesus fasted, He "was led by the Spirit into the wilderness" (Lk. 4:1). So it was with Elijah. Before his forty-day fast began, he was fed with angels' food. It sustained him during the forty-day fast as he journeyed through the wilderness on his way to meet with God.

So he arose, and ate and drank; and he went in the strength of that food forty days and forty nights as far as Horeb, the mountain of God (I Ki. 19:8).

As the forty days and nights drew to a close, he came to Mount Horeb. There he saw a mighty wind, experienced an earthquake and saw a fire. Then came the "still small voice" of God and a new anointing. Great as Elijah had been before, the new Elijah was greater. The new Elijah didn't run from anyone. Never again did he fear Jezebel and her wrath.

One of Elijah's first acts after his encounter with God was to return to Israel to anoint his successor, Elisha (I Ki. 19:16,19). Not long after that, Elijah pronounced judgment on Ahab and Jezebel for the murder of Naboth (I Ki. 21).

Fasting revolutionized Elijah's life. It gave him faith to meet Ahab and denounce the sins of the notorious Jezebel. It gave him faith to stand against all enemies. When the messengers of the king came to take him, he said, "If I am a man of God, let fire come down from heaven and consume you and your fifty men" (II Ki. 1:12).

Fasting gave him faith to promise Elisha that if he saw him at the time of his translation he would receive a double portion of his spirit. It gave him faith to get into the heavenly chariot and be caught away into heaven without seeing death. Fasting broke the spell of the one fear of his life — Jezebel. Fasting made him a conqueror, so that his influence was not only felt in that generation, but in all generations to the present day.

NINEVEH SAVED BY A FAST

The story of Jonah is familiar to all Bible readers. The lesson ordinarily preached is that those who attempt to flee from God find that sooner or later He catches up with them. This is a truth that can hardly be overemphasized. But there is another truth that is not often noted: It has to do with why Nineveh was spared the judgment the prophet proclaimed against the city.

Jonah was a runaway prophet. He foolishly boarded a ship bound for Tarshish to flee from the presence of the Lord. His experience in the fish's belly taught him a lesson. He obeyed the voice of the Lord and went to Nineveh to warn its residents of impending judgment.

And Jonah began to enter the city on the first day's walk.
Then he cried out and said, "Yet forty days, and Nineveh shall be overthrown!" (Jon. 3:4).

Things certainly looked bad for Nineveh. The prophet of God was boldly crying out in her streets that in forty days she would be destroyed. No doubt, the instruments of divine retribution had already been fashioned. Judgment hung suspended, as it were, by a thread over the capital of this Assyrian empire — the greatest city of that day. Warnings of divine judgment were not taken lightly. Other great cities such as Babylon, Tyre and Sidon, once among the greatest cities of the world, had fallen in accordance with the word of prophecy. Nineveh was also doomed.

However, God does not take pleasure in the death of the wicked. He is eager to delay or forego judgment if He can do it in a way that is compatible with divine justice. True repentance will turn away the rod of wrath. The king of Nineveh knew this. He believed the prophet's warning that catastrophe was at hand. He sent a proclamation throughout the land for the people to repent in sackcloth. All should fast and pray earnestly to God so that the city might be spared.

So the people of Nineveh believed God, proclaimed a

fast, and put on sackcloth, from the greatest to the least of them. ... But let man and beast be covered with sackcloth, and cry mightily to God; yes, let every one turn from his evil way and from the violence that is in his hands. Who can tell if God will turn and relent, and turn away from His fierce anger, so that we may not perish? (Jon. 3:5,8,9).

Many people call on God when they are in trouble. But those who are willing to fast until they receive an answer show that they are in earnest. As a result of Nineveh's people fasting and crying out to God, the Lord changed His mind and did not punish them.

Then God saw their works, that they turned from their evil way; and God relented from the disaster that He had said He would bring upon them, and He did not do it (Jon. 3:10).

ESTHER SAVES HER NATION THROUGH FASTING

The book of Esther is unique: The name of God is not mentioned once. But nowhere in the Bible is the providence of God more in evidence. This book tells the story of how Haman the Agagite planned to destroy the Jewish race. Through his scheming he managed to ingratiate himself with the king and persuaded him to sign a document authorizing the execution of all Jews living in the kingdom. The king was tricked and became an unwilling tool in the conspiracy. Too late he learned of the trap he had been led into. Mordecai, Queen Esther's uncle, brought the bad news to her, asking her to intercede with the king for their people. Esther reminded her uncle that if she entered the presence of the king uninvited, she jeopardized her life unless he held out the golden scepter. But Mordecai warned her that she would not escape death if she held her peace, though God would bring deliverance for the Jews through another source.

For if you remain completely silent at this time, relief

and deliverance will arise for the Jews from another place, but you and your father's house will perish. Yet who knows whether you have come to the kingdom for such a time as this? (Es. 4:14).

Esther made her decision. She told Mordecai to gather together the Jews in Shushan to enter into a fast with her and her maidens. Afterward, she would go in to the king.

Go, gather all the Jews who are present in Shushan, and fast for me; neither eat nor drink for three days, night or day. My maids and I will fast likewise. And so I will go to the king, which is against the law; and if I perish, I perish! (Es. 4:16).

The outcome of this fast was that Haman's wicked plans to destroy the Jews were thwarted. The gallows that were made for Mordecai were used to hang Haman and his sons.

Esther recognized that her most powerful weapon in a critical hour was to enter into a fast. She called her people to fast with her, which they did for three days and nights. Although it is not stated, we may be sure that they, like Jehoshaphat of old, cried mightily unto the Lord. The historian Josephus wrote:

Accordingly Esther made supplication to God after the manner of her country, by casting herself down upon the earth, and putting on her mourning garments, and bidding farewell to meat and drink and all delicacies, and she entreated God to have mercy upon her, and make her words appear persuasive to the king (Anti. XI, Chapter 6:8).

EZRA'S TRIP TO JERUSALEM

Ezra was among those who returned from Babylon to Jerusalem a few years after Cyrus' proclamation granting permission for the Jews to return to Israel. Some wonder why such a small number returned at that time. One reason was the thieves which populated the desert between Babylon and Jerusalem. They were willing to commit murder for small sums of money. Few dared to cross the desert unless accompanied by a large detachment of soldiers for protection. When Ezra and his companions chose to make the trip, they realized that their lives would be in grave danger. Ezra was a conscientious priest. He had assured the king that his God was the God of the whole earth. He felt that his testimony to the king would be weakened if he took a band of soldiers with them. Yet he knew the trip was hazardous. He thought of the wives and children whose lives would be in peril. What should he do? Ezra did the only thing he knew to do. He called for prayer and fasting:

> Then I proclaimed a fast there at the river of Ahava, that we might humble ourselves before our God, to seek from Him the right way for us and our little ones and all our possessions. For I was ashamed to request of the king an escort of soldiers and horsemen to help us against the enemy on the road, because we had spoken to the king, saying, "The hand of our God is upon all those for good who seek Him, but His power and His wrath are against all those who forsake Him." So we fasted and entreated our God for this, and He answered our prayer (Ezra 8:21-23).

Having completed their fast, Ezra and his companions began their journey. They brought much gold and silver along — a rich prize to the roving bands of thieves that infested the desert country. But the hand of God was with them and protected them from enemies that were waiting along the way. They finally reached Jerusalem safely, where they delivered the gold, silver and treasure to the temple.

ISRAEL SAVED FROM THE PHILISTINES THROUGH FASTING

There are other passages in the Old Testament that teach the value of fasting. One of these is found in I Samuel 7. The Israelites had gone through some sad experiences, including their loss of the ark of God to the Philistines. It had been restored, but the Philistines were again gathering against them. Samuel called on the people of Israel to forsake their gods and to turn from their sins. He called for a national day of fasting and prayer. In their distress, the people obeyed Samuel and said to him, "Cease not to cry to the Lord for us that he will save us out of the hand of the Philistines" (I Sam. 7:8). So the Lord thundered from heaven against the Philistines. They became confused and fled in panic. The Philistines never came again against Israel in the days of Samuel's leadership (vs. 10-13).

JOEL'S WARNING TO CALL A FAST AS THE DAY OF THE LORD APPROACHES

The prophet Joel takes us ahead by the Spirit of prophecy to the great day of the Lord. He sees it as a day of destruction. "Blow the trumpet in Zion, and sound an alarm in my holy mountain" (Joel 2:1), he cries as he perceives judgment approaching. Looking to the north he sees a great armed confederacy invading the land of Israel. It is a dark hour. What can be done? Joel has the remedy:

> Consecrate a fast, call a sacred assembly; gather the elders and all the inhabitants of the land into the house of the LORD your God, and cry out to the LORD. Alas for the day! For the day of the LORD is at hand; it shall come as destruction from the Almighty (Joel 1:14,15).

This is the day of the Lord, the hour of reckoning. What should be done? Again, Joel repeats: "Call a fast!"

> "Now, therefore," says the LORD, "Turn to me with all your heart, with fasting, with weeping, and with mourning." So rend your heart, and not your garments; return to the LORD your God, for He is gracious and merciful, slow to anger, and of great kindness; and He relents from doing harm. Who knows if He will turn and relent, and leave a blessing behind Him — a grain offering and a drink offering for the LORD your God? Blow the trum-

pet in Zion, consecrate a fast, call a sacred assembly;
gather the people, sanctify the congregation, assemble
the elders, gather the children and nursing babes; let the
bridegroom go out from his chamber, and the bride from
her dressing room" (Joel 2:12-16).

That is the message of the prophet Joel. If the people will humble
themselves and truly repent, God will drive away the northern
invader. More than that, He will pour His Spirit out upon all flesh
and "whoever calls upon the name of the LORD shall be saved"
(Joel 2:28-32).

Chapter 6

Triumph Over the Prince of Persia

Daniel is another remarkable character in the Bible. He lived for a century, much of that time employed in a high government office. On several occasions, his life and those of his friends were placed in jeopardy because of their open faith in Jehovah God. Once Daniel was thrown into a den of lions, and on another occasion his three friends were tossed alive into a fiery furnace. But on each occasion, God gave miraculous deliverance.

Daniel survived several regimes and changes in government. Successive rulers recognized the merits of the prophet and honored him with great responsibilities in the kingdom.

When Daniel was in his last years, he was not as active in affairs of state as he once was. But he was as active as ever in the ministry of intercession. In Ezekiel 14:14, Daniel is mentioned along with Job and Noah as men who had unusual favor with God. Daniel knew the mighty power of prayer. Three times a day he knelt and lifted up his voice in praise to God in worship. This daily habit of the prophet is mentioned in connection with his persecution at the time he was thrown into the lion's den.

> Now when Daniel knew that the writing was signed, he
> went home. And in his upper room, with his windows
> open toward Jerusalem, he knelt down on his knees three

times that day, and prayed and gave thanks before his
God, as was his custom since early days (Dan. 6:10).

The secret of Daniel's success was that he prayed his way
through life. The result of his prayer was that God was with him.
Though the powers of darkness time and again rose up against him,
the Lord gave him supernatural deliverance on every occasion.

DANIEL PRAYS AND THE CAPTIVITY COMES TO AN END

One of Daniel's great victories in prayer warfare is recorded in
Daniel 9. On this occasion he was reading the writings of Jeremiah,
which declared that Israel's captivity was to last 70 years. Consult-
ing the calendar, the prophet saw that the time was up. The over-
throw of the Babylonian Empire had just taken place. Daniel entered
into deep intercession. He fasted and prayed that God would fulfill
His promise to restore the Jews to their land.

Then I set my face toward the Lord God to make request
by prayer and supplications, with fasting, sackcloth, and
ashes (Dan. 9:3).

Prostrate before God, the prophet confessed the sins of his
people. While he was praying, the angel Gabriel was dispatched
from heaven to tell him what would happen to his people. The angel
reassured Daniel that the commandment would go forth "to restore
and to build Jerusalem" so that his people would flourish once again
in their homeland. He also gave Daniel the wonderful prophecy of
the coming of the Messiah.

Know therefore and understand, that from the going
forth of the command to restore and build Jerusalem
until Messiah the Prince, there shall be seven weeks and
sixty-two weeks; the street shall be built again, and the
wall, even in troublesome times (Dan. 9:25).

What a wonderful victory this was! Within a short time, Cyrus
issued the "commandment" authorizing the Jews to return to Jeru-

salem (see Ezra 1:1-3).

THE 21-DAY FAST

This revelation from the angel about the Messiah made Daniel's burden for his people increase. The Messiah was to come, but the prophecy declared that He was to "be cut off!" (Dan. 9:26). What would be the fate of his people after that tragic event took place? The matter weighed so heavily upon Daniel that he determined to pray and fast until the answer came. And the story of this great 21-day intercession is told in Daniel 10-12.

> In those days I, Daniel, was mourning three full weeks. I ate no pleasant food, no meat or wine came into my mouth, nor did I anoint myself at all, till three whole weeks were fulfilled (Dan. 10:2,3).

The inference from the words he "ate no pleasant food" is that he received slight nourishment. At any rate, he set himself before God in prayer, determined to get an answer. Previously the answer had always come quickly. Daniel probably did not realize on the first day of his intercession that three whole weeks would go by before he would have his answer. But that is what happened! For 21 days he wrestled in prayer with seemingly no indication that any answer was on the way.

Apparently others were with him during this time, sympathetic with his intercession for his people, but understanding little of spiritual warfare. For on the twenty-first day when the answer came, the supernatural manifestation which accompanied the appearing of the angel so alarmed them, "they fled to hide themselves" (Dan. 10:7).

The effects of the 21-day fast were felt by the aged prophet. He said that "no strength remained in me; for my vigor was turned to frailty in me, and I have retained no strength." However the touch of the angel apparently strengthened him (verses 8,10).

THE ANGEL EXPLAINS A MYSTERY

The angel addressed Daniel saying, "O Daniel, man greatly beloved" (vs. 11). What a salutation! Men today scheme and strive for position in the kingdom of God, but promotion and honor from God are not obtained that way. It is given to the intercessors and prayer warriors who do not war with flesh and blood but who unflinchingly war against the spiritual forces of darkness.

The angel then explained the mystery of the delayed answer. He told Daniel that on the first day he had set himself to obtain an answer from God, his words had been heard and the angel sent to him:

> Then he said to me, "Do not fear, Daniel, for from the first day that you set your heart to understand, and to humble yourself before your God, your words were heard; and I have come because of your words" (Dan. 10:12).

Now comes the most revealing information in the Bible concerning the operation of the forces of darkness — a power which dominates the kingdoms of this world, resists the saints and even resists the very angels of God. This is one of the most remarkable revelations of the Old Testament. It gives us a unique glimpse into what takes place above us in the unseen world. The "prince of Persia" was not the human ruler of Persia; he certainly had no power to resist an angel. It was no doubt a spirit prince under Satan.

The fact is, there is a spiritual kingdom composed of principalities and powers. Each nation has its unseen spirit ruler. Each earthly kingdom is under the sway of organized forces of wickedness which seek to bend it completely to their will. That this present evil world is almost completely under the dominion of Satan, is clearly revealed in Luke 4:5,6:

> Then the devil, taking Him up on a high mountain, showed Him all the kingdoms of the world in a moment of time.

And the devil said to Him, "All this authority I will give You, and their glory; for this has been delivered to me, and I give it to whomever I wish."

Under Satan there are subordinate princes, who in turn have armies of demons under them. All of them work toward one purpose: to bring all the intelligences of this planet under the devil's control. Those who believe that man is evolving from a lower species and that in time a super-race will come forth which will create its own millennium, are under the grossest kind of delusion. Human attempts at race regeneration are hopelessly impotent. Only the preaching of the Gospel can have any effect in changing man's fallen nature.

Spiritual powers in high places are dislodged only by spiritual warfare. The strength of the "prince of Persia" is realized in the fact that for three weeks he was able to successfully hinder the angel from getting through to Daniel. Only when God sent reinforcements by the Archangel Michael did the powers of darkness at last give way.

This "prince of Persia" highly resented his authority being disturbed, and fiercely resisted intrusion into his domain. Nevertheless, Daniel continued praying, and his prayer aided in releasing the spiritual power needed to defeat the powers of darkness.

What would have happened if Daniel had given up? The answer is obvious. Daniel's faithfulness in prayer determined the outcome of the struggle in the heavenlies. Because he persisted in prayer, the "prince of Persia" was defeated.

There is a great lesson here for us on how to obtain answers to prayers that seemingly are not being answered. Note that no mysterious providence of God prevented the answer. Those who do not want to pay the price of "praying through" sometimes make the excuse that God is not answering because He knows they would be better off with their prayer unanswered. The reason some prayers are not answered is simply because there are active evil powers in the world that resist the saints receiving answers to their petitions.

The devil and his demons cannot be everywhere at once, nor successfully prevent the answer to all prayers. Therefore, they determine who of God's saints are doing the most harm to the kingdom of darkness at the moment and concentrate their efforts against them. Evil powers sometimes prevail only because God's people do not understand the hindering power of Satan. Paul once said that he had planned to minister to the Church of Thessalonica, "but Satan hindered us" (I Thes. 2:18).

The devil's power *is* limited. The shield of faith will quench all the fiery darts of Satan. Persistent battling in prayer will ultimately result in routing out the enemy. God will, if necessary, dispatch an archangel to the assistance of the man or woman who is faithful in prayer. And if the enemy continues his assaults and more reinforcements are necessary, God has additional resources. He will send all the help that is needed. Christ said to His disciples as He faced the cross:

> Do you think that I cannot now pray to My Father, and
> He will provide Me with more than twelve legions of
> angels? (Matt. 26:53).

We must not forget the place that fasting plays in all this. For three weeks, "no pleasant food" came into Daniel's mouth. For three weeks he continued in travail of soul, wrestling against the forces of darkness. He did not know that an angel had been dispatched to bring him the answer. He prayed on in faith, stubbornly refusing to accept failure, believing that surely the answer would come. And so it did.

The answer was not only good, it was wonderful. The Lord revealed the things Daniel wanted to know about the destiny of his people in the years to come. He also showed the prophet what would take place at the end time. The angel took him to the days of the great tribulation and showed him the signs that will then take place. "Until the time of the end; many shall run to and fro, and knowledge shall increase" (Dan, 12:4). He showed him the rise of the Antichrist, who will enter and destroy many countries. Daniel was shown how this self-willed king will magnify himself against the God of gods, but finally "come to his end, and no one will help him" (Dan. 11:45).

Having revealed all these things, the angel showed Daniel that when the time of trouble reaches its worst, God Himself will come and raise the dead, reward the righteous and judge the wicked.

> At that time Michael shall stand up, the great prince who stands watch over the sons of your people; and there shall be a time of trouble, such as never was since there was a nation, even to that time. And at that time your people shall be delivered, every one who is found written in the book.
>
> And many of those who sleep in the dust of the earth shall awake, some to everlasting life, some to shame and everlasting contempt. Those who are wise shall shine like the brightness of the firmament, and those who turn many to righteousness like the stars forever and ever. But you, go your way till the end; for you shall rest, and will arise to your inheritance at the end of the days (Dan. 12:1-3,13).

Shouldn't we, like Daniel, be intercessors? Shouldn't we desire to be "greatly loved" by God as Daniel was? Shouldn't we hold on by prayer and fasting until the answer comes? If so we persevere like the prophet did, we too "shall rest, and will arise to your inheritance at the end of the days."

Chapter 7

Fasting in the New Testament

ANNA THE PROPHETESS

One of the first characters introduced in the New Testament is Anna the prophetess. She was nearly a century old and lived in the temple, fasting and praying and waiting upon God.

> And this woman was a widow of about eighty-four
> years, who did not depart from the temple, but served
> God with fastings and prayers night and day (Lk. 2:37).

Perhaps there were those who wondered what she had accomplished in all those years. But it is evident that her prayers played a part in preparing the way for the coming of the Messiah. When the Christ-child was brought into the temple by Joseph and Mary, the Spirit revealed His presence to her. So it was with inexpressible joy that she gave thanks before the people that this was He Who would bring redemption to Israel — the Redeemer she had been looking for so long.

CHRIST IN THE WILDERNESS

Christ, the perfect man as well as the Son of God, began His ministry with a forty-day fast. Perhaps we will never know all that was accomplished by this fast, but we may be sure that it played an important part in the preparation of the Lord for His redemption ministry.

Before going into the wilderness, Jesus was baptized in water by John the Baptist in the River Jordan. He was also filled with the Holy Spirit. Then the Spirit led Him into the wilderness.

Then Jesus, being filled with the Holy Spirit, returned from the Jordan and was led by the Spirit into the wilderness (Lk. 4:1).

Observe that Christ was filled with the Spirit before He began the fast. Two things are revealed here: First, one may fast and be helped by it (as the heathen seamen fasted with Paul on board the ill-fated ship that was destroyed in the storm), but the baptism of the Spirit is needed to fast to the greatest advantage. Second, when the Holy Spirit comes, He will lead His people to fast, though probably not for forty days, except in rare instances. There will be times in every Christian's life when the Spirit will lead him to fast.

What did Christ do during those forty days in the wilderness? He met the full impact of Satan's power and temptations.

And He was there in the wilderness forty days, tempted by Satan, and was with the wild beasts; and the angels ministered to Him (Mk. 1:13).

We see from the experience of Christ that one of the purposes of fasting is to give men power over the temptations of the flesh. Think of the multitudes of Christians still in bondage to the flesh. They are oppressed with habits and complexes that take away their victory and leave them defeated and powerless. Many of these people are sincere and earnest, but their flesh is so powerful that they see no way to break the chains which bind them. Some have tried everything, seeking a solution to their difficulties. Many times they have turned over a new leaf or made new resolutions. But in the end, they have looked in the face of failure.

There is a solution for bondage to the flesh. "However, this kind does not go out except by prayer and fasting" (Matt. 17:21).

Satan came to Jesus in the wilderness and said, "If You are the Son of God, command that these stones become bread" (Matt. 4:3). After fasting for forty days, Christ was surely hungry. But He would not make bread for the devil. Later, He multiplied the loaves and fish until there was enough to feed a multitude.

Again Satan came to Christ and tempted Him. He took Him to the summit of a high mountain and "showed Him all the kingdoms of the world in a moment of time. And the devil said to Him, 'All this authority I will give You, and their glory; for this has been delivered to me, and I give it to whomever I wish'" (Lk. 4:5,6). Christ indignantly rejected Satan's offer. He did not want to reign over the devil's kingdom. The hour would come when He would reign as King of kings and Lord of lords, but not until the kingdoms of this world become the kingdoms of our Lord Jesus Christ.

Next Satan took Christ to the pinnacle of the temple and told him to prove His divinity by casting Himself to the ground. In this temptation of the soul, the devil quoted Scripture which promised that the angels of God would bear God's people up, "lest you dash your foot against a stone" (Lk. 4:11). But Jesus, having no intention of putting God's power on display for the mere purpose of creating a sensation, replied, "It has been said, 'you shall not tempt the LORD your God'" (Lk. 4:12). Later Christ would overrule the power of gravity by walking on water as a sign to His disciples.

Through those days of fasting in the wilderness, Christ overcame every temptation, whether it affected His body, spirit or soul. And we must remember that Christ was both divine and human, and "was in all points tempted as we are" (Heb. 4:15). Therefore, we too can master temptations of body, soul or spirit through prayer and fasting.

THE TEACHING OF CHRIST CONCERNING FASTING

That Christ intended His disciples to fast is evidenced by His teaching. He did most of His fasting before He began His active ministry. The Pharisees were always looking for some complaint against Jesus. On occasion, they called attention to the fact that John's disciples often fasted, yet they had never seen Christ fast. The Lord did not enlighten them by telling them that He had fasted forty days at the beginning of His ministry. If they wanted to be ignorant, they could be ignorant. He *did* give the reason why He did not ask His disciples to fast while He was with them. He plainly said that after He was taken away, they would fast.

> Then they said to Him, "Why do the disciples of John fast often and make prayers, and likewise those of the Pharisees, but Yours eat and drink?" And He said to them, "Can you make the friends of the bridegroom fast while the bridegroom is with them? But the days will come when the bridegroom will be taken away from them; then they will fast in those days" (Lk. 5:33-35).

While Christ was present, His power and presence caused evil powers to flee. If the disciples failed, the Lord was at hand to deliver. But after He was gone, it would be necessary for them to advance into the place of dominion that He lived in. To do so, fasting would be necessary.

The truth of this is brought out in the case of the epileptic boy whom the disciples could not heal. Though they tried to cast the devil out in the name of Jesus, this stubborn evil spirit held his ground and refused to move. Then Christ came on the scene and showed there was no reason that the boy could not be healed. Speaking with authority, He cast out the evil spirit. Afterward, the disciples came to Him and asked, "Why could we not cast him out?" (Matt. 17:19). Jesus' answer shows some circumstances, problems and demons cannot be dealt with effectively without fasting and prayer.

> So Jesus said to them, "Because of your unbelief; for assuredly, I say to you, if you have faith as a mustard seed, you will say to this mountain, 'Move from here to there,' and it will move; and nothing will be impossible for you. However, this kind does not go out except by

prayer and fasting" (Matt. 17:20,21).

Fasting combined with prayer is the key to mastery over the impossible.

Chapter 8

Fasting in the Early Church

The most important conversion in the early Church was associated with a fast — that of the Apostle Paul. The apostle, by his own testimony, had been a blasphemer and was an accessory to the death of the first martyr, Stephen. Paul had seized men and women because of their faith, and had them thrown into prison. In his last act of persecution, he had secured letters from the high priest for the purpose of uprooting the church at Damascus. But as he approached the gates of the city, the Lord Jesus appeared to him in a vision of dazzling brilliance. The astonished young Pharisee asked what he should do. He was commanded to go into the city, where he would be told what to do. Blinded by the vision, the apostle had to be led into Damascus. He immediately began a fast. For three days he did not eat or drink anything.

> And he was three days without sight, and neither ate nor drank (Acts 9:9).

At the end of the three days, God spoke to Ananias, one of the Christians in Damascus. He told him to go and lay hands on Paul that he might receive his sight and be filled with the Holy Spirit "for behold, he is praying" (Acts 9:11). Ananias did not want to go at first, but the Lord explained what had happened — that Saul had seen a vision of Ananias "coming in and putting his hand on him, so that he might receive his sight" (Acts 9:12).

God could have sent Ananias the first day, but He did not. Those three days of prayer and fasting prepared Paul for his deliverance. People who have serious afflictions would do well to pray and fast like Paul until they have the assurance for the answer. If a person's faith is too weak to secure deliverance on his own from some chronic affliction, he might be completely healed if he would pray and fast before hands were laid on him by a minister of the Gospel.

FASTING OPENED THE DOORS OF THE GENTILES TO RECEIVE THE GOSPEL

Cornelius was a godly man, a centurion "who feared God with all his household, who gave alms generously to the people, and prayed to God always" (Acts 10:2). He had not yet received the message of salvation through Christ, but his soul was crying out to God for a full revelation of His will. He was praying and fasting one day, and at about three o'clock in the afternoon, an angel suddenly appeared before him. The angel told him that his prayers and works of charity pleased God. He told Cornelius to send for Peter (his location and name were given) and Peter would tell him about the way of salvation.

In the days of the apostles many religious people prayed. What was it about Cornelius' prayer that pleased God? No doubt God was pleased with his deep sincerity. But we must not forget that his prayer was accompanied by fasting — a vitally important factor. When Peter arrived at his house, Cornelius said,

> Four days ago I was fasting until this hour; and at the ninth hour I prayed in my house, and behold, a man stood before me in bright clothing, and said, "Cornelius, your prayer has been heard, and your alms are remembered in the sight of God" (Acts 10:30,31).

While Peter preached about "how God anointed Jesus of Nazareth with the Holy Spirit and with power, who went about doing good and healing all who were oppressed by the devil" (Acts 10:38), the Holy Spirit came and fell on Cornelius and his whole household. Fasting without sincerity will accomplish nothing, as was the case with the Pharisees. But fasting and praying in sincerity is powerful; it moved heaven for Cornelius. In this case, it opened the door for the gentiles to receive the Gospel.

FASTING PRECEDED THE FIRST MISSIONARY ENTERPRISE

The time came when the call of God to reach the unevangelized began to weigh heavily on the hearts of Paul and his companion, Barnabas. They had been ministering in the church at Antioch. Paul remembered how the Lord had spoken through Ananias at Damascus, saying that Paul was to be sent on a mission to the gentiles. Considerable time had now elapsed, yet Paul had never gone to the gentiles, nor had the Lord made it clear how or where he was to go. Now he and Barnabas, as well as some of the others, thought it was time to obtain the answer from God. So they decided to enter into a fast:

> As they ministered to the Lord and fasted, the Holy Spirit said, "Now separate to Me Barnabas and Saul for the work to which I have called them" (Acts 13:2).

How many days were spent in this fast we do not know, except that they stayed before the Lord until the answer came. God could have given them specific directions without the fasting, but He did not. There was a reason why a fast was in order. A spiritual battle needed to be waged and won against the powers of darkness so that when they went out on the field, the way would be open before them. As they ministered to the Lord, the answer came: Set aside Paul and Barnabas for the work God had called them to do.

One might think that having received divine instructions, the apostles would have left immediately. But they did no such thing. Now that they knew what the Lord wanted them to do, they desired the blessing of God on their plans more than ever. So it was that the whole church fasted and waited on the Lord before a move was made. Finally, hands were laid on Paul and Barnabus and they were sent on the world's first missionary journey.

Their first stop was in Cyprus. The Spirit of God moved right from the start. Even the interest of the proconsul of the country, Sergius Paulus, was stirred. He called for the apostles because he wanted to hear the Word of God. But Elymas, the sorcerer, used his influence to try to turn the proconsul away from the faith. Because of those days of fasting in Antioch, Paul was ministering under a powerful anointing. Suddenly, he looked straight at the magician and rebuked him, informing him that judgment was coming on him for a time. Immediately Elymas was struck blind. The proconsul, astonished by what had happened, became a believer.

The first stage of this historic missionary journey was a great success. No doubt this success came because their ministry had been preceded by prayer and fasting. Without the supernatural power which came because of the fast, it is possible that the apostles would have left Cyprus frustrated and defeated instead of victorious and triumphant.

Chapter 9

A Twenty-Three-Day Fast for Revival

by Len Jones

The following is the story of a 23-day fast by Col. Len Jones, a former chaplain in the Australian armed forces. We believe this day-by-day account of the fast by this Australian editor and evangelist will give much information and insight into the proper way to fast. It will also show some of the results of such a fast.

This is a diary of a 23-day fast. There is one thing God has against fasting, and He has the same against prayer and almsgiving, and that is that we do it "to be seen of men," and to glory in what we do before others. For that reason I am hesitant in putting the experience on paper. But as I read the Scriptures of the many testimonies of fasting, I am made to feel it is God's will for this experience to be made known. That convinces me that there is a place in which we can give fasting testimony, not to receive honor from men, but to bring blessing to others.

This was a complete fast. No food was taken during the fast. Only water was taken. During the time of the fast, I was conducting evangelistic meetings every night except Monday, and two meetings on Sunday. I remained in South Africa one year, and during that time thousands knelt at the altar for salvation, restoration, healing and consecration of their lives afresh for the service of the Lord.

THE NEED IN SOUTH AFRICA — CAUSE OF THE FAST

When I arrived in South Africa, the whole union opened up to me for evangelistic campaigns, but I felt totally inadequate for the situation. I was conscious of a tremendous spiritual need — first, for a much deeper experience with God myself, and second, for a ministry for this country.

Something had to be done! The need was desperate! I was brought up against a brick wall — unless God met me I knew I would be a failure. Praying alone did not seem to make the slightest impression upon the burden — I could see no other way out but to fast and pray. It was a call of God! It was my only hope!

I did not know how long I would fast — I did not make a decision. I have found it wiser to start that way, for if you make a time and do not continue until that time, there can be a sense of frustration that might mar a little of the great blessings received.

1st Day — Hardest of All

Everything was black and hopeless! It was a miserable day! The first day is generally the hardest of all. Most of the day was spent in prayer — such conditions often lead you to prayer.

2nd Day — First Blessing Received

Today I felt brighter in spirit and more confident. I was not very hungry, but drank quite a lot of water. It is good to drink plenty of water while fasting. I felt weak, but this is exactly as I expected for this is generally such during the first three days of fasting, and explains why Jesus said when He fed the four thousand, "I have compassion on the multitude, because they have now been with Me three days, and have nothing to eat: And if I send them away fasting to their own houses, they will faint on the way: for divers of them came from afar" (Mk. 8:2,3 KJV).

During the day I was very conscious of the presence of the Lord and His blessing and peace, and in the early hours of the morning had a mighty time with God in prayer. The Lord gave me faith that all the many things being prayed for would be answered — this was a wonderful and powerful time of intercession.

3rd Day — Weakness Felt

I felt weak this morning, as was to be expected. My tongue was coated and there was a bad taste in my mouth. In the afternoon, I walked about four miles, visiting and praying. In the evening I had a wonderful meeting with the power of God in evidence.

4th Day

This evening had a wonderful meeting, when the subject was "Faith." The whole congregation was at the altar for prayer. Let me say here that if this time of prayer and fasting were stopped right now, the services we have been having, have been more than worth it all.

5th Day — Weakness Begins to Leave

Today I was very bright in spirit and body. The feeling of weakness and lassitude that I have had during the first few days has gone and I feel fine.

The meeting in the evening was best yet. Who says that fasting as well as praying is not abundantly worthwhile?

6th Day — Blessings Increase

As I awoke this morning I felt better and stronger than I have since I started fasting.

Today is Sunday and I have two meetings. What a wonderful meeting it was this morning. Right from the start the presence and power of God was on the meeting. Without invitation many came to the front for prayer. Physically, I felt a lassitude and weakness today with the long meetings. But with it all I felt so restful and peaceful with a steady confidence in God.

7th Day — Prayer Necessary

Today I realized afresh it must be fasting and prayer, and not fasting alone. Both are necessary!

At the end of the first week I weighed myself and found that I had lost about twelve pounds, which is about right. You lose much more the first week than later. As the fast proceeds it generally works out at a loss of weight of about one pound a day.

8th Day — Some Physical Reaction

When I awoke this morning there was more physical distress, but it is this that constrains you to prayer. There was a feeling of dizziness but the blessings were wonderful. There was such a peace and confidence and I felt I had such a grip of things — I felt I could meet anyone with ease and with authority. In the spirit, also, all was well — it seemed that I had vacated from the natural into the spiritual and it was wonderful.

And after all, the physical inconvenience should be expected. The natural must decrease while the spiritual increases. Daniel did not have an easy time with his 21-day fast. Scriptu.e says he was in mourning the whole time (Dan. 10:2). Daniel says, "There remained no strength in me: for my comeliness was turned in me in corruption, and I retained no strength" (Dan. 10:8 KJV). (Also read experience of the Psalmist, Psalm 109:23-25.) And so it is with us! But Daniel and David had a wonderful spiritual experience.

Today I start a campaign in another church, and had to go stay with new people. One of the biggest trials in fasting is the people with whom we live, especially those who love us and are dear to us — they get so concerned about us.

The tendency to quit came over me this morning. "The Lord had blessed and answered my prayers. Perhaps this is enough." In the afternoon I felt so much brighter and wondered why I had ever considered ending the fast. There are moods and changes in fasting. Watch and pray!

9th Day

This was a busy day and I was on my feet most of the morning. Feeling very well in body and happy in the Lord. Preached with much blessing tonight.

10th Day — Self-examination

Just as my body has been objecting to the elimination of toxins, poisons, accumulated waste matter and other things that offend, and bids me to stop the fast, so now I am finding my spirit is objecting to the elimination of things that are displeasing to God, and bids me quit.

This is a fight to the death of everything in me (spiritual and physical) that is contrary to the will of God. And what a fight it is. How the spirit is resisting. There is no mistaking it when God shows you yourself — it takes away all your self-righteousness all right. What a fight is going on as these things lift their ugly heads, but they have to go in the same way as things that offend physically have to go.

In a time of prayer and fasting you see yourself as others see you and as God sees you. This affords you an excellent opportunity to confess and deal with all such things. As the fasting continues I am expecting other things to come up — I am also expecting that they will be dealt with.

11th Day

All is going well spiritually and physically. I feel that I am taking a vacation in heaven. Physically there is nothing like the discomfort there was a week ago. Many others are being blessed and encouraged to fast and pray. A great work has been done. Tonight, feeling that the fast has served a wonderful purpose there is a strong desire to cease. But not only am I prepared to cease I am prepared to carry on if that is God's plan.

12th Day — New Strength Comes

Today has been a very easy day. All who have fasted, testify of the feeling of weakness, nausea and lassitude that you have the first few days and which continues up to the first week. All goes as you get around the twelfth and thirteenth day. In fact, and I know that only those who have fasted will believe me when I say it, around the fourteenth day you actually get stronger as the time goes on.

13th Day — Selfishness Revealed

Today the Lord has been dealing with me again about greed, covetousness and selfishness. As I have seen myself I seem to have been such a selfish person, always concerned about my interests — interests in God's work, yes, but also very much interested in my own needs and comforts. What a time I have had this morning! I have been low before the Lord! And then there is another great battle, closely allied to pride — wanting to be somebody in the eyes of men, wanting to impress, a hesitance to take an humble place, and being more concerned with what man thinks of your ministry than what the Lord thinks. And so these two battles were fought today in intense earnestness, with a keen desire that my heart shall be laid bare before God and that a new experience will be my portion.

What a time we had in the meeting last night, and again this morning. Many testified of healing as a result of prayer for them last night. Oh that people would pray and fast — what a difference it makes, both in regards to our own lives and ministry. It is worth it a thousand times and brings blessings that nothing else can bring.

14th Day

Today I was on my feet all through the day until 4 p.m. How well and strong I feel! It is always unbelievable that one actually gets stronger when they pass into the third week. Only those who have experienced it will believe it! To others it must sound like exaggeration. But how well in spirit one feels, for this time of prayer and fasting is primarily a consecration fast unto the Lord.

A week ago in the morning, as I packed my suitcase in preparation for a move to this present home, I was very weak. As I packed I had to sit down and rest, but tonight, although at the end of a very busy day, there is no feeling of weakness. It is simply amazing.

17th Day — Great Faith Being Born

Today I feel wonderful. Fasting is no trial now, and the days come and go beautifully and easily. Spiritually I feel that I am in another world. It is a wonderful experience and the end is not yet. I believe as the fast continues I am going to get to that place with God that my soul has been longing. A man came to the house today to be prayed for with pains in the stomach. I felt such faith as I put my hands on him. He was healed instantly and went away rejoicing. This is happening continually in the meetings night after night.

18th Day — Healing Ministry Being Developed

This was not such a good day. I went to the meeting with the conviction that I had not sought God sufficiently this day — yes, it is to be prayer as well as fasting. But as soon as I started to preach all tiredness left me. After I had prayed for many sick people I felt better than I had felt all day. It was encouraging tonight to hear about a dozen testify that they were healed when they were prayed for the night before.

19th Day

Today I had an attack in my body of a trouble from the days in the army, probably through army food and conditions. I am glad that it came up at this time as it enabled me to do some real praying about it.

20th Day — Increasing Blessing

What wonderful meetings we are having. A great crowd gathered last night in the city hall. Many testified in this morning meeting of instantaneous deliverance from all kinds of troubles.

Today I preached in a way that I have seldom preached before. I seemed to have faith to believe for almost anything. Well, we are fulfilling the conditions: "Nothing shall be impossible unto you. Howbeit, this kind goeth not out but by prayer and fasting" (Matt. 17:20,21 KJV). When you are fasting, you feel that you have done the last thing and there is nothing more you can do — it seems to give you a claim on God for the supernatural to happen.

Everyone is rejoicing at the blessing and presence of the Lord in our midst. Never do I remember being so completely concerned about the will of God only! Never did everything outside God's will seem so uninteresting and uninviting.

21st Day

One of the purposes of this fast was to encourage others to fast and pray, and to convince by example that no bodily harm would result. As people see me preaching night after night, looking little different than when I started, it is inspiring many others to fast and pray.

23rd Day — Fasting Ends

The appetite we have for food is very often from habit, and is not a true habit but a perverted one. Just like a heavy smoker would rather have a smoke than a meal — he has an appetite, a very real appetite, for it, but it is not a true need. This false appetite for food goes after about three days. It is not till many days later that the real appetite comes.

It is then that fasting finishes and starvation begins. This is the time to cease. It is at this time your tongue clears, your mouth and breath sweeten, and weakness returns. That is why we read about Jesus, "And when He had fasted forty days and forty nights, he was afterward an hungered" (Matt. 4:2 KJV), which suggested that He had not been hungry before.

Two or three days ago, I remarked about a new color in my face and today my tongue, mouth and breath are sweet. And with this I have a ravenous hunger. For this reason I have decided this afternoon to finish my fast. ... Weighing myself at the close of the fast, I found I weighed 149 pounds compared to 176 pounds at the beginning, or a loss of 27 pounds in twenty-three days.

BREAKING THE FAST

It is obvious that after so long without food, the utmost care must be taken in breaking the fast. This cannot be over emphasized — the longer you fast, the more care must be exercised. Impatience here can cause much harm!

It is good to break such a fast as this with fruit juices diluted one to three — any fruit juice will do, but orange juice is best. The first day take a half glass of orange juice diluted with water, three or four times during the whole day. Double this amount the second day (it is best to take it warm). The third day drink the orange juice undiluted. Perhaps a little fruit may be taken. On the fourth day you can take several meals of fresh fruit. On the fifth day take a half pint of milk every two hours. On the sixth day you can begin eating meals of raw vegetables such as tomatoes, carrots and lettuce. From now on you can gradually work back to your usual diet.

Breaking your fast is more difficult than the fast itself. You will certainly be a very unwise person and will risk serious damage, which could prove fatal, if you unduly rush this breaking of the fast period.

With all my heart I thank God for the past twenty-three days. Words fail to express the blessings I have received both spiritually and physically, and I believe the results of the fast which follow will be even greater than the results during the fast have been.

SPECIAL NOTE: A free gift subscription to CHRIST FOR THE NATIONS magazine is available to those who write to Christ For The Nations, P.O. Box 769000, Dallas, TX 75376-9000. This magazine contains special feature stories of men of faith and includes prophetic articles on the latest world developments. Why not include the names of your friends? (Due to high mailing rates, this applies only to Canada and the U.S.)

Christ For The Nations
International Missions

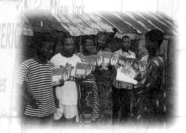

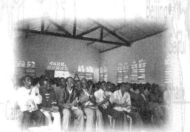

Literature Program

International Bible Schools

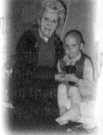

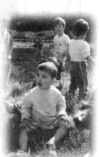

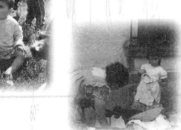

Support to Orphans

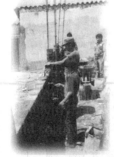

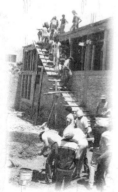

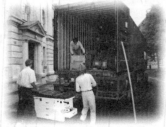

Native Church Program

Humanitarian Aid & World Relief

CHRIST FOR THE NATIONS
P.O. Box 769000 • DALLAS, TX 75376-9000
1-800-933-2364 • www.cfni.org

Life-changing Intimate Worship

Christ For The Nations
INSTITUTE
Prepare For Your Destiny

Dynamic Teaching Of The Word

Taking It To The World

Advanced schooling is available in missions, pastoral, and worship & the arts.